THE DANGERS OF HERBAL STIMULANTS

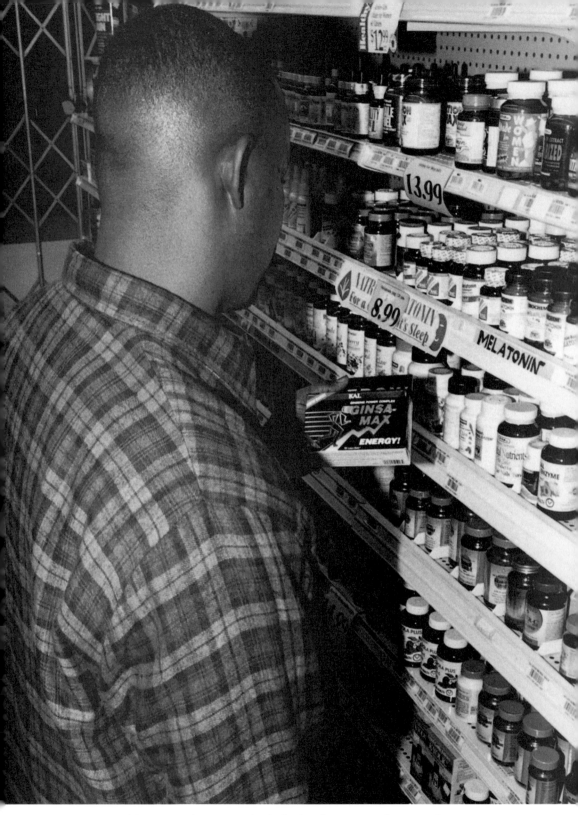

Many people assume herbal stimulants are safe to use because they are legal and made with natural herbs.

THE DRUG ABUSE PREVENTION LIBRARY

THE DANGERS OF HERBAL STIMULANTS

Meish Goldish

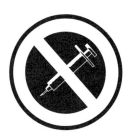

THE ROSEN PUBLISHING GROUP, INC.

NEW YORK

The people pictured in this book are only models; they in no way practice or endorse the activities illustrated. Captions serve only to explain the subjects of the photographs and do not imply a connection between the real-life models and the staged situations shown. News agency photographs are exceptions.

Published in 1998 by The Rosen Publishing Group, Inc.
29 East 21st Street, New York, NY 10010

First Edition

Library of Congress Cataloging-in-Publication Data
Goldish, Meish.
    The dangers of herbal stimulants / Meish Goldish.
        p. cm. — (Drug abuse prevention library)
    Includes bibliographical references and index.
    Summary: Explains the different types of herbal stimulants as well as dangers and benefits associated with their use.
    ISBN 0-8239-2555-2
    1. Herbs—Toxicology—Juvenile literature.
    2. Stimulants—Toxicology—Juvenile literature.
    [1. Herbs. 2. Stimulants.] I. Title. II. Series.
    RA1250.G65   1998
    615.9'52—dc21   97-6986
                                                       CIP
                                                        AC

Manufactured in the United States of America

Contents

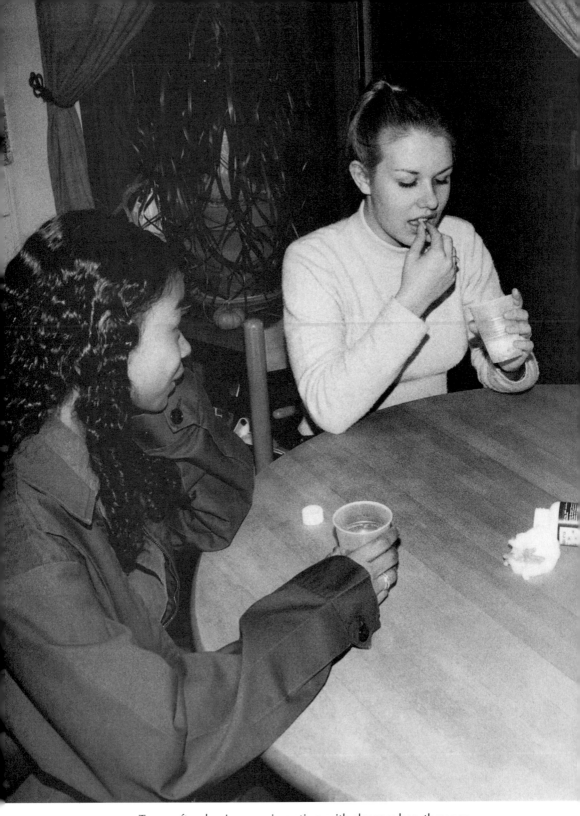

Teens often begin experimenting with drugs when they are hanging out with friends.

CHAPTER 1

Peter and Kristina

*P*eter came from Long Island, New York. He was a popular teenager. Everyone in school seemed to know him.

One year Peter planned a vacation. He went with some friends to Florida. He and his friends shared a motel room near the beach.

On their first day, the group went downtown to check out the beach town's main strip. Some of the shop windows had large ads for pills called Herbal Ecstacy, Cloud 9, and Ultimate Xphoria. Peter had never heard of them. But the ads made them sound exciting. They promised users euphoria, increased energy, mood elevations, inner visions, and sexual sensations.

8

Peter asked about the pills. The store clerk said they were legal and didn't cost a lot. He also said they were made of natural herbs, so they weren't bad for you.

It sounded like safe fun. Peter and his friends decided to try Ultimate Xphoria. The package said to take four pills at a time. But the store clerk suggested taking twelve to fifteen for a real high.

Back in the motel room, Peter's friends each took a dozen pills. Peter was a little afraid. So he only took eight. Soon he got a bad headache. His legs and arms tingled. That night he told his pals to go out without him. When they returned, Peter was dead. Later, doctors said he died from a mixture of caffeine and an herb called ephedra. Both are stimulants that speed up the heart. And both are ingredients in Ultimate Xphoria.

Why did Peter die but not his friends? Every human body is different. Some people can handle certain substances more easily than others can. But Peter isn't the only person to die from Ultimate Xphoria. In the United States, at least seventeen people have died from it or from other stimulants like it.

Kristina lived in San Jose, California. For several weeks, she hadn't been feeling well. Finally she visited her doctor. He told her she was pregnant. Kristina was very upset by the news. So was her boyfriend. They both felt they couldn't afford to raise a child at this point in their lives.

Kristina wanted an abortion, but she was scared to go to the doctor. One of her girlfriends had had one. But her friend told her the operation had been awful. The doctor was not friendly. He didn't seem to care about his patient.

She spoke with another friend. She learned about an herbal stimulant that could abort (end) a pregnancy. It was called Fresh Pennyroyal Herb. It could be taken in the privacy of your room. Best of all, it was legal and was sold in health-food stores.

Kristina bought some Fresh Pennyroyal Herb. The package didn't say what the product was for. But she followed the directions exactly.

One night, soon after Kristina began taking the mixture, she became very ill. She felt sharp, stabbing pains in her stomach. She began to sweat a lot. After a while, she passed out. Her boyfriend found her later, still unconscious.

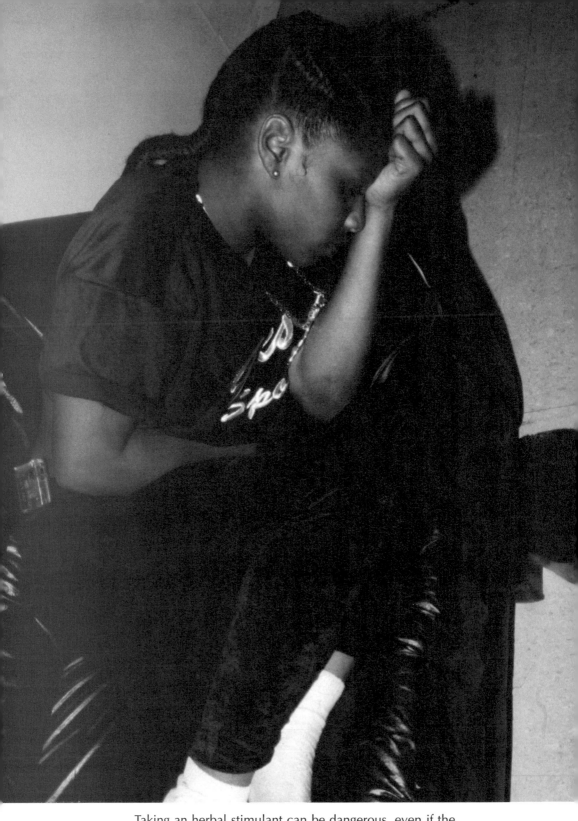

Taking an herbal stimulant can be dangerous, even if the directions on the package are followed exactly.

At the hospital doctors removed the
dead fetus. It had settled in Kristina's fal-
lopian tube. That caused a lot of bleed-
ing. Kristina bled so much she went into
shock and died. Doctors said that the
shock was caused by abnormal blood
clotting from liver damage. The liver
damage had been caused by pennyroyal.

Kristina's parents were very angry.
They believed that pennyroyal had killed
their daughter. Her parents sued the herb
company for damages. They also asked
that a warning be placed on all future
pennyroyal packages produced by the
herb company.

More than a dozen other women have
died after taking pennyroyal for abortions.

You may have learned that because
something is herbal, it is safe. But Ultimate Xphoria and Fresh Pennyroyal Herb
are two herbal stimulants that can have
dangerous results. They are sold legally in
stores. More than 100 companies in the
United States make herbal products. Are
they all dangerous? If so, why are they
legal? What are the risks of taking herbs?

Types of Herbal Stimulants and Their Dangers

*S*timulants are chemicals that speed up or increase the activity in a part of the body.

Many stimulants speed up the brain. Caffeine is an example. It is found in coffee. That is why tired drivers sometimes drink coffee. It helps them stay alert.

Some illegal drugs contain stimulants. Amphetamines are an example. They are sometimes called speed or uppers. The chemicals make the heart beat faster. Amphetamines can cause heart attacks, strokes, and death.

Some herbs contain stimulants, too. In Chapter 1, you read about ephedra. Its chemicals, plus caffeine, are what killed

Peter. They stimulated his heart until it simply gave out.

Herbal stimulants can be deadly. But not in every case. It depends on how the herbs are used in products. And how those products are used by buyers.

Today stores sell many herbal stimulants. One of the most powerful is ephedra. Products with ephedra can be placed into three main groups:

- Products for getting high
- Products for fitness
- Products to help breathing

Herbal Ecstacy

These pills first appeared in 1992. The maker is Global World Media Corporation in Los Angeles. The company is headed by Sean Shayan.

Herbal Ecstacy is very popular. It is sold in dance clubs, record stores, and sex shops. Between 1992 and 1996, about 150 million pills were sold. Sales exceeded $300 million.

Ads for Herbal Ecstacy call it "the world's first 100 percent natural, organic (without chemicals), legal, and safe alternative to a harmful, illegal recreational chemical."

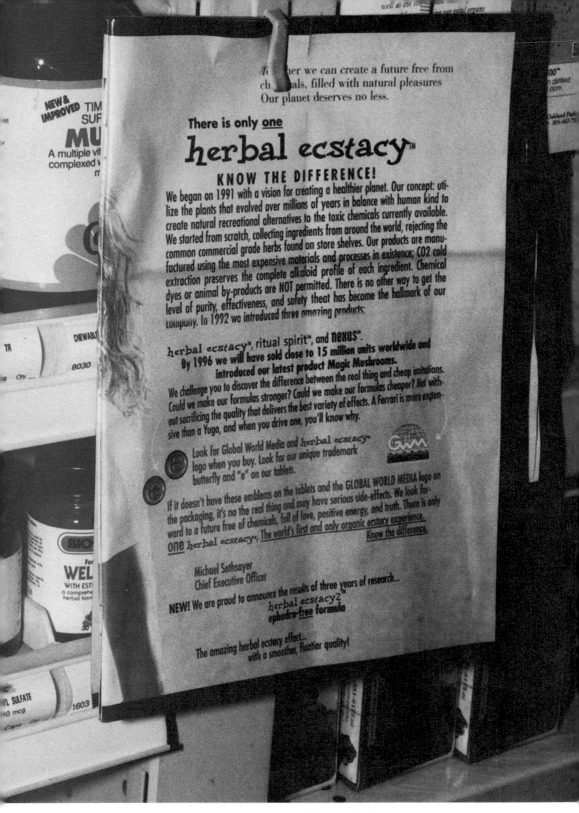

Herbal Ecstacy was created to offer a "safe" alternative to the illegal drug Ecstasy.

Many experts don't agree. They say it is not safe. They say it can be as harmful as an illegal drug.

The main ingredient in Herbal Ecstacy is the herb ephedra. The Chinese call it *ma huang*. For thousands of years, it has been used to cure asthma and allergies. It contains two chemicals: ephedrine and pseudoephedrine. They stimulate the heart, blood vessels, and brain. Today the same chemicals are used in popular cold medicines like Contac and Sudafed.

When used properly, ephedra can help breathing. But the makers of Herbal Ecstacy discovered something else. Mixed with caffeine, it can give users a high. Within twenty minutes, a user's heart rate and blood pressure jump. Herbalists at Shayan's company experimented. They mixed ephedra with other herbs that contain caffeine. The result was Herbal Ecstacy.

Herbal Ecstacy is a powerful stimulant. It's especially dangerous for anyone with high blood pressure, heart disease, or diabetes. It is not a drug. But it acts very much like one. Some people call it an imitation drug. Others call it nonprescription speed.

16   Even the name Herbal Ecstacy
suggests that it is a drug. It is named
after Ecstasy (the last *s* has been
changed to *c*). Ecstasy is a dangerous,
illegal drug that works like LSD. It has
different effects on different people. It
makes users hallucinate. They hear
and see things that aren't there. Some
users feel sick and vomit. At least a
dozen people have died from taking
Ecstasy.

Herbal Ecstacy doesn't have the same
ingredients as Ecstasy. But it too can be
harmful. The same goes for another of
Shayan's herbal stimulants, Magic Mushrooms. It is named after an illegal drug,
psilocybin mushrooms. The two products are not the same. But the herbal
version can be just as unsafe as the
drug.

Other Highs

Herbal Ecstacy is a popular product. It
has led to many spin-offs. Companies
now make other herbal stimulants for
getting high. They include Ultimate
Xphoria, Cloud 9, Euphoria, Herbal
Bliss, Rave Energy, Brain Wash, and
Buzz Tablets. All contain ephedra and
caffeine. And all can be dangerous.

More than 400 users have reported bad reactions to those stimulants. They include insomnia, dizziness, nausea, memory loss, and muscle injury. They also include high blood pressure, liver failure, strokes, heart attacks, and nerve damage.

Other herbal stimulants have been associated with health problems. These include Black Lemonade, Brainalizer, Fungalore, Herbal XTC, Hextasy, Legal Weed, Naturally High, Planet X, the Drink, and X Tablets.

In January 1997, forty-two people in their teens and early twenties were hospitalized after drinking vials of herbal liquid products at a New Year's Eve dance concert in Los Angeles. The products were made by Biolife Bioproducts and contained the ingredient Kava Kava. People suffered from severe shortness of breath, nausea, and respiratory arrest. One seventeen-year-old had a heart attack. The Food and Drug Administration (FDA) issued a warning on the products, variously known as Cherry fX Bomb, Orange fX Rush, and Lemon fX Drop. Many of the people had taken a much higher dose than what was suggested on the package.

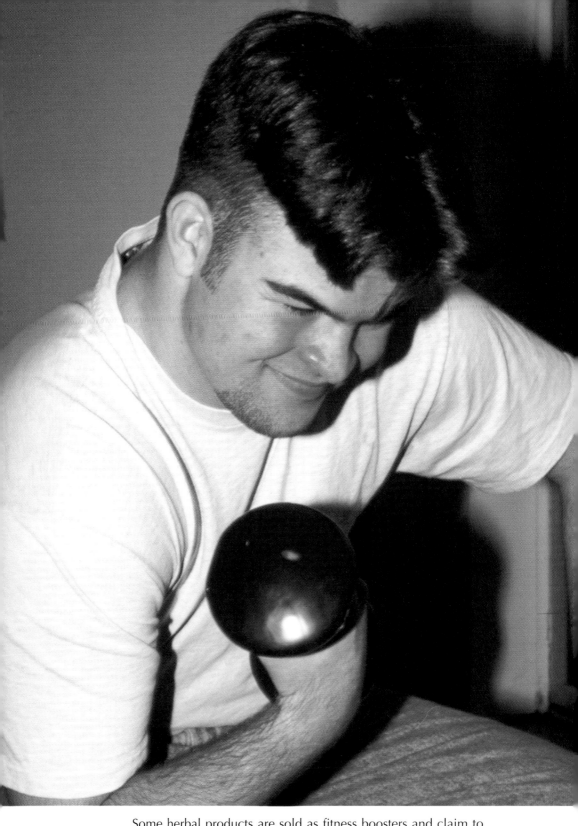
Some herbal products are sold as fitness boosters and claim to build muscles and increase energy.

The Role of the FDA

The FDA was established in 1928. It is an agency that regulates all foods and drugs. The FDA needs to approve any product before it can be sold to the public. It can also stop the sale of any food or drug that it determines unsafe. Some drugs are so safe that many are sold without a prescription. They come with complete instructions and warnings on the packages. But they should only be *taken as directed*. Otherwise they could also do harm.

Fitness Products

Some herbal stimulants are not aimed at drug users. They are for health and fitness fans. They aren't sold at dance clubs or sex shops. Rather, they're found in health-food stores, drugstores, and supermarkets.

These ephedra products are for losing weight, building muscles, boosting energy, or increasing sex drive. They have names like Ripped Fuel, Blasting Caps, and Up Your Gas.

But like the herbal products for getting high, the fitness boosters contain ephedra. So are they as dangerous as stimulants like Herbal Ecstacy?

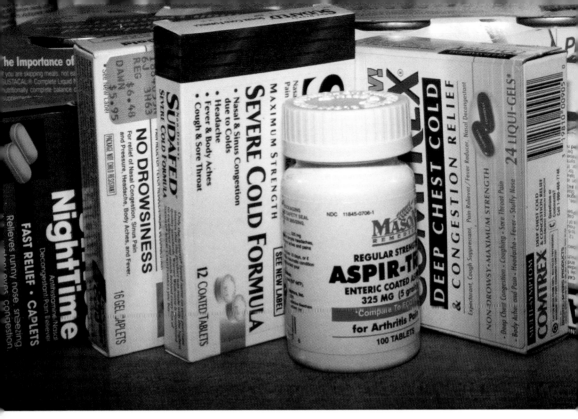

Many medicines in drugstores contain small amounts of the same herbs found in herbal stimulants.

Makers of the fitness products say no. Some have been selling them for fifty years or more. They say their products are much safer than those used for getting high. They use lower amounts of ephedra. They offer more information on package labels.

It's true that fitness products are not the same as those for getting high. But they still can be risky. You should *never* start using any product with ephedra on your own. It should only be taken with a doctor's approval and supervision.

Breathing Products

The third group of ephedra stimulants are those to help breathing. They include medicines for allergies, colds, flu, and asthma. They are sold in drugstores and supermarkets.

Stimulants in this group are the safest to take. They have been approved as safe drugs by the FDA.

Other Herbal Stimulants

Today stores sell many other kinds of herbal stimulants in addition to ephedra. They come in the form of pills, liquids, powders, tablets, tinctures, teas, and creams. They can be bought without a prescription. Here is information on some of them.

Belladonna

This herb is also known as deadly night-shade. It is a poisonous plant. Even so, its chemicals are found in some prescription drugs for asthma, colds, and hay fever. In small doses, belladonna can be useful. But in larger doses, it can be deadly. In the 1990s at least seven people have been poisoned by tea made with belladonna leaves.

22 | ## *Chaparral*
People have used this herb to treat skin problems, ease arthritis, prevent cancer, and slow the aging process. But in 1992 the FDA warned that chaparral could cause liver damage. In 1995 the FDA reported fifteen cases of people getting liver disease from taking chaparral.

Coltsfoot
Scientists disagree about the safeness of this herb. It contains large amounts of vitamin C. Many doctors in Germany consider it a good cure for coughs and breathing problems. But other doctors disagree. In Japanese lab tests, coltsfoot caused cancer in rats.

Comfrey
This herb was originally placed on the skin to reduce swellings of boils, bruises, and sprains. Some users now take it orally for stomach ulcers and arthritis. But comfrey, when swallowed, can damage the liver by depriving it of blood.

Echinacea
This herb is used widely to treat colds and flu. In Germany, it is injected into patients. In the United States, a pill is

swallowed. Some people find the herb bad tasting, but it has no known side effects. Doctors warn not to use echinacea for more than a week at a time.

Germander

This herb is commonly found in tea and tablet form. It is sold more in Europe than in the United States. It is advertised as a diet product. But it has been blamed for at least twenty-seven cases of hepatitis.

Ginger

Women in China drink ginger tea to relieve menstrual cramps and morning sickness. In America, ginger ale is a popular stomach soother. Research has shown that taking ginger before a trip can prevent motion sickness.

Ginkgo

This herb has been used to treat memory loss, headaches, ringing in the ears, impotence (the inability to get an erection), and depression. In Germany, ginkgo is prescribed often. Doctors consider it safe if taken in small amounts. But large doses can cause restlessness, stomach upset, diarrhea, and vomiting.

24 | ## Ginseng
This herb has been promoted as a cure for everything from stress to poor memory to diabetes. One popular ginseng product is Ginsana. Ads say Ginsana will help build energy and endurance. But scientific studies have found little proof of that. Taking too much ginseng can cause nervousness, insomnia, and diarrhea.

Lobelia
Native Americans used lobelia as a healing herb. At one time it was approved by the FDA as a drug to cut down on smoking. Today it is found in some herbal products to ease muscle spasms and to help digestion. But it is no longer claimed to help people quit smoking. Taking too much can cause vomiting, breathing problems, rapid heart rate, sweating, and even coma and death.

Pennyroyal
This herb has many uses. Some people rub the leaves on their bodies to keep away fleas and mosquitoes. Others breathe the herb to treat coughs and menstrual cramps. It has also been taken in liquid form as a way to induce

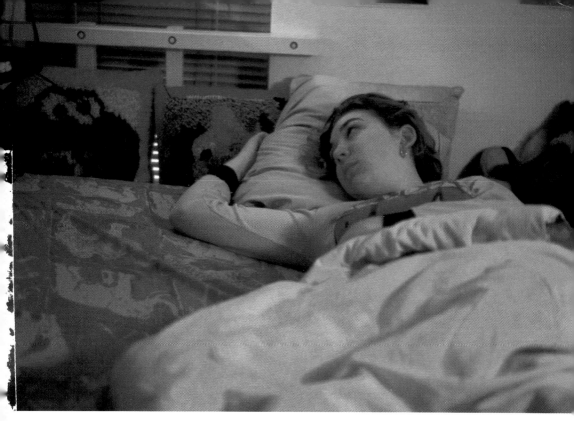

Taking certain herbs over a long period of time can result in serious illness.

abortion (see Chapter 1). But in liquid form, pennyroyal can be very dangerous. It can cause liver damage, convulsions, coma, and death.

Sassafras

Native Americans once drank sassafras tea as a cure for fevers, spasms, and syphilis (a sexually transmitted disease). Later, the roots of the herb were used as flavoring in root beer. But in the 1960s, tests showed that sassafras caused liver cancer in rats. In 1970 the FDA banned sassafras as a food additive. Today some

26 | people still use the herb to relieve the itch of poison ivy.

Senna

For more than a thousand years, people have used this herb as a laxative, a product to relieve constipation. It is found in many laxatives sold today. Senna is also drunk by some as a diet tea. The FDA says senna is safe if taken only occasionally and in small amounts. Long-term use can lead to heart problems.

Yohimbe

This herb is advertised as a body builder and sex booster. But it can be very dangerous because it raises blood pressure. The FDA says yohimbine, a chemical found in yohimbe, is unsafe. An overdose can cause weakness, seizures, paralysis, kidney failure, and death.

CHAPTER 3

Teenagers and Herbal Abuse

*T*eenagers take herbal stimulants for different reasons. Many do it to get high. Some do it to try to stay fit. Some do it to relieve medical problems.

For the careful user, herbal stimulants do little or no harm and may even be beneficial. But for those who abuse them, they can be harmful, even deadly.

What can happen when teens abuse herbal stimulants? Here are some actual cases.

"I Want to Get High"

Rosanna was a teenager who loved to party. On Fridays, she would go to all-night dances. There she would take the

28 | drug Ecstasy to get high. But one time she took a bad dose. She spent the entire night vomiting. "I thought I was going to die," she said.

Then Rosanna heard about Herbal Ecstacy. She thought it would be safer than Ecstasy. Her first time, she took ten pills. Within a half hour, her heart started pounding wildly. She fainted three times. She was rushed to the hospital. Her stomach had to be pumped. Doctors told her she almost died.

"I'm Too Fat"

Rachel felt she needed to lose weight. Her doctor and parents didn't agree with her. But that didn't change Rachel's mind. "My friends are all thinner than me," she said.

Rachel heard about an herbal diet tea. It was made with senna. She bought some at a health-food store. She drank it for four months. She lost some weight. But one night she fainted. She was rushed to the hospital. Doctors said the tea had been destroying her body. It was robbing her of potassium. Potassium is needed to regulate the heartbeat. The tea caused Rachel serious heart problems.

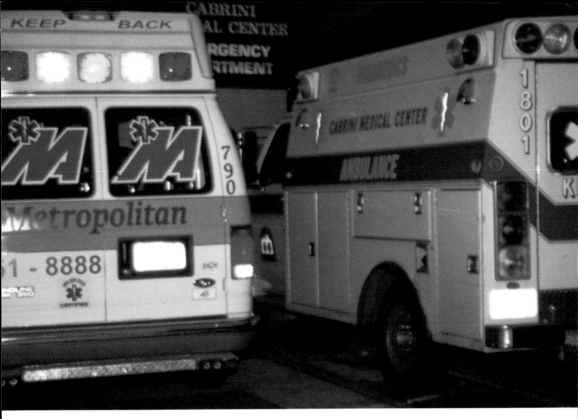

Some people intentionally take a larger dose of an herbal stimulant than is suggested and must be rushed to the hospital.

"I Want Muscles"

Darrell was on his high school wrestling team. He was in good shape. But he wanted to further build his muscles. He knew that steroids were dangerous. His coach had warned him about them.

In a health-food store, Darrell found a sports-training formula. It contained ephedra. For a few months, Darrell took two pills daily before working out. One morning he had a stroke during his work-out. It caused permanent brain damage. His doctor said the ephedra formula caused his stroke.

"I Need Energy"

30 | Chanice often felt tired in school and at home. She rarely ate healthy foods. She stayed up late. But she didn't want to have to change her bad habits.

Then a friend told her about the herb Siberian ginseng. Her friend said it was a great energy booster. Chanice started taking large doses every day. It gave her the energy she wanted. But after a while she started to feel dizzy. While driving home one day, she had an accident. She didn't know that Siberian ginseng contains pure grain alcohol. By using this herb, Chanice was practically drunk every day.

"It's Great for Sex"

Gary began having sex when he was fourteen. His friends bragged of "doing it all night" after taking special tablets. They contained the herbs yohimbe and Korean red ginseng. Gary wanted to try them.

Gary began taking the tablets. He thought they would help him maintain an erection longer. Instead, he couldn't get an erection at all. Gary had low blood pressure. Yohimbe causes impotence for people with this condition. It made Gary feel anxious and depressed.

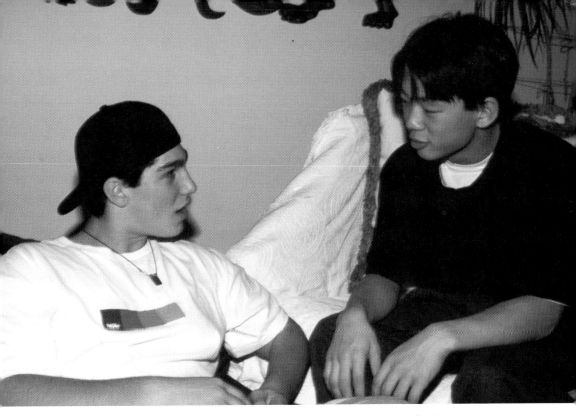

Friends can be a strong influence on the decisions you make in your life.

"I've Got Cramps"

Teresa often got painful monthly cramps. She tried over-the-counter drugs sold in the drugstore. But none helped very much.

A friend said that the herb chaparral could ease cramps. Teresa began to take it. At first it helped her. But after a few months, it caused her diarrhea and stomach pains. Teresa did not stop taking the chaparral. Instead, at her friend's suggestion, she increased her dosage. In time, it led to serious liver damage.

31

32 | ## "My Friends Do It"

Nick went to a school where lots of students do drugs and herbal stimulants. On weekends, his friends sometimes took yohimbe for a sex high. Nick had never heard of yohimbe. But his friends said, "It's herbal, so it's okay."

Nick tried some at a party. He also had some red wine and cheese that night. Later his skin broke out in an ugly rash. So did his friends'. They didn't know that yohimbe should not be taken with foods, such as wine and cheese, containing tyramine, an amino acid. The combination can cause bad rashes.

Questions About Stimulants

Every year more teenagers are tempted to try herbal stimulants. Many new users have questions about the products. You may have some, too. Here are the answers to some questions often asked.

Are They Safe?

It depends. If you're talking about stimulants for getting high, no. Products that mix ephedra and caffeine are very dangerous. They can cause heart attacks, strokes, and seizures. They can also cause death. They are especially dangerous for

people with high blood pressure, heart
disease, or diabetes.

33

Products used for fitness purposes also
carry risks. Some companies that make
them are not very reliable. Their products
may contain bad formulas. There may be
few warnings or directions on the labels.
The products might contain ingredients
that are impure or contaminated.

Remember that most herbal products
do not require testing by the FDA. As a
result, you can never be sure what's in a
package. Sometimes an herb is misidenti-
fied when picked. Belladonna, a poisonous herb, can easily be mistaken for
parsley. Sometimes two packages of the
same product can contain different
amounts of herbs—or different herbs
altogether.

Herbal products with FDA approval are
marked "FDA Approved" and are the
safest to use. That's because the ingredients have already been tested. Always
check the package first. Never assume
that because a product is for sale, it's
been approved by the FDA.

Are They Good for You?
Many people think that herbs are always
good for them. That is not always true.

34 | Hemlock and belladonna are herbs. They are also poisonous. Arsenic and strychnine are some chemicals found in herbs. They, too, are poisonous.

Some herbal stimulants may be good for you in small amounts, but not in higher ones. One or two cups of coffee a day can be a pick-me-up with few or no side effects. But five cups a day can cause headaches and nervousness. Much more than five can cause dizziness, ringing in the ears, and temporary hearing loss.

Some herbs may be healthy in one form, but not in another. Pennyroyal is an example. Its crushed dried leaves can be rubbed on the skin to keep insects away. But pennyroyal *oil* can be deadly. If swallowed, it can kill.

An herb may also be good for some people, but not for others. Many herbs are harmful to women who are pregnant or nursing a baby and to people with high blood pressure, heart disease, or diabetes.

Never think that since it's herbal, it's good. Find out from a doctor how healthy the herb is for *you*.

Do They Really Work?

It depends. If you're looking to get high, you may be disappointed. Some teens

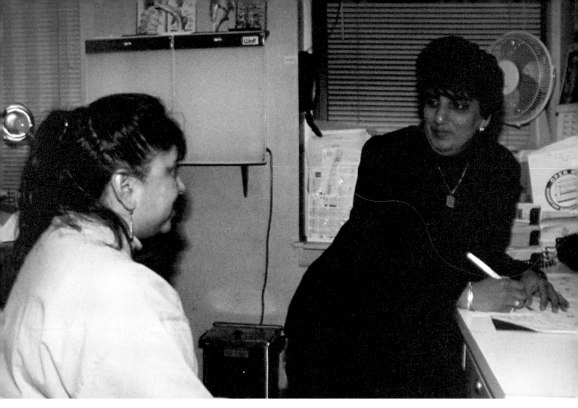

If you are thinking about trying an herbal stimulant, talk to someone about it before you do it.

swear they get high. The stimulants may work for them. But that doesn't mean they will work every time or that they are safe. One bad dose and the user could be dead.

Do fitness products work? That also depends. A diet aid may work for one user, but not for another. Why? Because every human body is different. Your body may respond to a certain chemical stimulant. Your friend's body may not.

Even medicines work differently for different people. You and a friend can take the exact same kind of cold

36 | medicine. Your cold symptoms may go away, but your friend's may not.

Are They Addictive?

Addictive means habit-forming. You probably know that many drugs, like heroin and cocaine, are highly addictive. After a while, users are not able to control or stop their drug use.

Herbal stimulants are not addictive in the same way that drugs like heroin or cocaine are. Those drugs are *physically* addictive. Users who try to stop can suffer body aches, diarrhea, muscle cramps, or nausea.

Many experts believe that herbal stimulants can become *psychologically* addictive. That means users *think* they need them to feel good.

As far as science now knows, herbal stimulants are not physically addictive. But users may develop a psychological dependence on them.

CHAPTER 4

A History of Herbs

*H*erbs are plants that are used as medicine. (They are also used to flavor food.) Use of herbs as medicine dates back to the earliest times. Long ago, people used herbs to cure aches, coughs, colds, sores, and more. They used the leaves, bark, flowers, fruits, and stems of plants. They found that the herbs worked. Herbal medicine became very popular in ancient China, India, and Egypt. Today it is still practiced by many people. Those who work with herbs are called herbalists.

Like other medicines, herbs affect your body and how it functions. Also like other medicines, herbs can help—or, when misused, can hurt—your body.

Nearly everyone in the world uses herbs. That includes you. In some

38 countries, herbs are still a main source of medicine. In the United States, some of our most popular foods and drinks come from herbs. You may not think of them as medicine. But long ago, other people did.

Coffee

Coffee is America's most popular herbal drink. Today most people use it as a mild stimulant or a pick-me-up. But in ancient Africa, men ate raw coffee beans before fighting or hunting. It made them feel strong and alert. Later, coffee was used for relief of asthma, fever, headaches, colds, and flu.

Today coffee is not considered a healing herb in most cultures. In fact, drinking more than a few cups a day can even be harmful. Coffee contains a powerful stimulant, caffeine. Too much can make you jittery. It can also become habit-forming, or addictive.

Tea

Tea is the most common herbal drink in the world. People in ancient China were probably the first to use tea as medicine. It has about half the caffeine found in coffee. Like coffee, it is drunk mainly as a mild stimulant. But tea is also used for

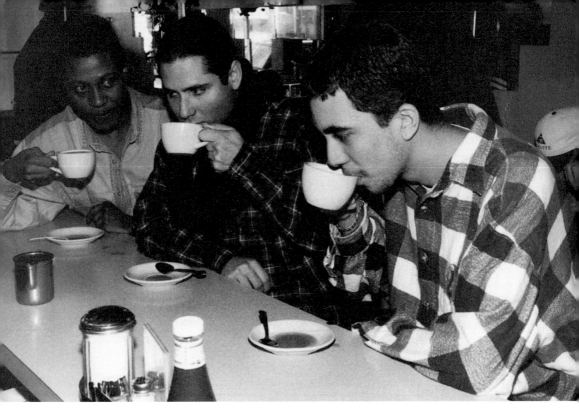

Every time you drink a cup of coffee, you are taking a mild herbal stimulant.

relief from diarrhea, colds, coughs, and breathing problems.

Today tea is still a popular herbal medicine. The Chinese even use it to treat hepatitis, a serious liver disease. Since tea has fluoride, it can also help fight tooth decay.

Soft Drinks

You probably don't think of today's soft drinks as herbal medicine. But some of their ingredients were originally used as herbal medicine. For instance, in the 1500s, the English made their own

40 stomach medicine with ginger. It was called ginger beer. We still drink a form of it today. It's called ginger ale.

Coca-Cola was first developed as a cure for headaches. It was invented in the 1880s by a pharmacist in Atlanta, Georgia. He made an herbal drink with kola nuts. Today some doctors recommend cola drinks for children with asthma.

Chocolate

Do you like chocolate? Then you like herbs. Chocolate, or cocoa, comes from cacao beans (the fatty seeds of a South American evergreen tree). In the 1500s, the Aztecs ate chocolate for its taste. But it had other uses as well. Central Americans drank cocoa for relief from fevers, coughs, and pregnancy pains. They rubbed cocoa butter on burns, chapped lips, and balding heads.

Today chocolate is mainly a sweet treat. But some people use it as a mild stimulant. It has about one-fifth the caffeine found in coffee.

Mints

Have you eaten peppermint candy? For a long time, mints have been an herbal medicine. They're listed in the world's oldest medical book, Egypt's *Ebers Papyrus*. It mentions mint as a stomach soother. Ancient Romans and Greeks ate mint after meals to help digestion. Herbalists used it for everything from hiccups to leprosy.

Today peppermint is still a popular stomach soother. It's used in medicines like Tums and Phillips' Milk of Magnesia. Herbalists also use peppermint oil on burns, scalds, and herpes sores.

Native Americans and Europeans

Europeans first came to America around 1500. Herbalists who arrived were very surprised to find that Native Americans also used many herbs for medicine. Some were the same herbs used by the ancient Chinese and Egyptians. The Native Americans were healthy and strong. So Europeans began to study their medicines. They learned about the healing powers of chaparral, wild cherry, witch hazel, and other herbs.

Things began to change in the 1700s. In the American colonies, doctors studied medicine at universities. They said that herbal medicine was not a true science. They thought it was not reliable.

42 | Herbalists felt the same way about modern medicine.

Herbs in Modern Times

In the 1900s medicine made much progress. As a result, herbal medicine became even less popular. American medical schools mostly ignored herbs. In pharmacies, herbal products were removed from the shelves. They were replaced by new drugs made with chemicals.

Not all the new drugs proved safe, however. Some were laced with alcohol, cocaine, and heroin. They harmed many users. The public demanded more safety. So in 1928 Congress took action. It established the Food and Drug Administration (FDA) to regulate and approve any product before it is sold to the public.

Since the 1950s the FDA has watched over medicine even more closely. All new drugs must be tested for safety before they can be sold. Testing one new product can cost a drug company up to $100 million.

But herbs are different. The FDA says they are not drugs or medicine. They are food supplements. So most herbs don't have to be tested for safety, as drugs do. They can be sold in drugstores and

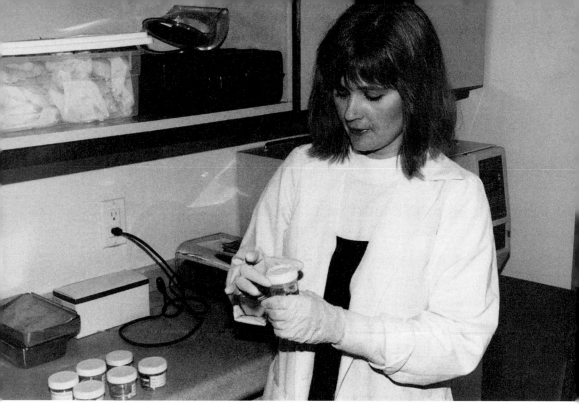

Any new drug must be tested for safety by the FDA before it can be sold.

health-food stores, often without prescription.

In recent years, the health-food business has boomed. From 1981 to 1991 the sale of herbs doubled to reach 1.3 billion dollars each year. By 1995 there were more than 8,000 health-food stores in the United States. Herbs like garlic, ginseng, chamomile, and ginger became best sellers. People took them to stay healthy and prevent illness. In 1995 sales for herbal supplements hit $2 billion.

The Drug Craze

44

A health-food craze began in the 1960s. But with it came another new craze— drugs. Many teenagers started taking amphetamines, also known as speed or uppers. In the 1980s crack and cocaine also became popular. All those drugs are stimulants. People took them to feel good, or get high.

But the drugs were very dangerous. Many users became addicted to them. The drugs were often deadly. And they were illegal. People faced fines and jail time for using or selling them.

The drug craze has continued into the 1990s. The death and danger also have continued. That is when herbs entered the picture.

In 1991 Sean Shayan, then 15 years old, was living in Los Angeles. He was a school dropout who worked at L.A.'s nightclubs. He watched teenagers go to all-night dances called raves. At the raves, many took an illegal drug called Ecstasy. It made them high and gave them energy to dance. The high could last for several hours. But when the high wore off, users felt awful and very depressed. The drug was dangerous. It was costly. And it was illegal.

Shayan had an idea. He thought about creating an alternative to illegal drugs. It would still be used for getting high. But it would be made with herbs. It would be all-natural, legal, and cheap.

Shayan's idea led to a new craze in the 1990s: herbal "high" stimulants.

CHAPTER 5

Herbal Stimulants and the Law

When Herbal Ecstacy first came out, ads said: "It's legal." Many teens were pleased by that. They knew that buying illegal drugs was risky. You could be arrested, fined, and sent to jail or prison.

But not with Herbal Ecstacy. It isn't sold illegally on the street. It is on the shelves of food stores and other shops.

But in recent years, many laws have changed. Is Herbal Ecstacy still legal? What about other herbal stimulants? This chapter will discuss new laws that have been passed recently.

In the Past
Since 1928 the FDA has controlled the drug industry. Each new drug must be

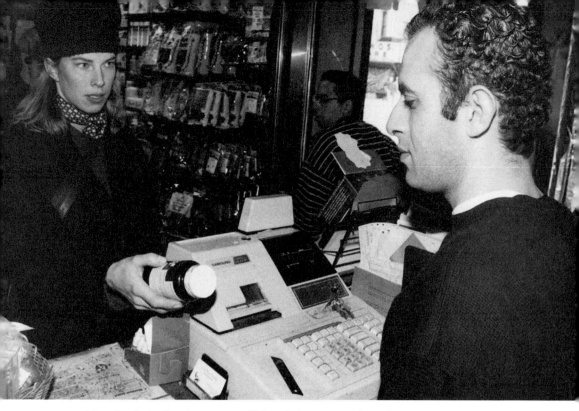

Most herbal stimulants are still legal, but recent laws have limited their availability.

tested before it can be sold as medicine. Makers must prove that the drug works and that it's safe.

But as we discussed before, the FDA has never considered most herbs to be medicine. So it does not treat them as drugs. It does not watch over the makers of herbal products as it does makers of other drugs.

A New Federal Law

In 1993 the FDA decided to look closer at herbs. It knew that some herbs had been

48 responsible for poisonings and deaths. The FDA wanted stricter laws for selling herbs.

That news concerned many herb users. They feared that their favorite herbs might be banned by the FDA. Millions of people wrote letters to Congress. They demanded that their herbal products be kept legal.

In 1994 Congress passed a new law. It was called the Dietary Supplement Health and Education Act. It put herbs, vitamins, and minerals into a special category: dietary supplements.

Here is what part of the 1994 law said:

- Supplements can be sold without being tested first to see if they work.
- Companies don't have to prove their supplements are safe. If the FDA wants to remove a supplement, it has to prove the product is unsafe.
- Supplement makers do not need to follow any one standard. That means the same product, made by two different companies, might have completely different ingredients.
- A package can make limited claims about a product. It can't claim to cure or prevent a disease. But it can

say how the product affects the body. **49**
For example, an herbal package cannot claim that the product cures
cancer. But it can say that it protects
against cell damage.

The 1994 law pleased both makers of
herbal products and users. That's because
the rules for herbs remained fairly relaxed, as before.

New State Laws

Not everyone was happy with the new
law, however. Many lawmakers felt it was
too relaxed. It did not ban the sale of
herbal stimulants that they believed were
dangerous.

As a result, some states took their own
action. They passed their own laws. For
example:

- In 1994 Ohio limited sales of ephedra products. They can be sold only
  by licensed pharmacists. Buyers must
  be at least eighteen years old.
- In 1996 Florida banned the sale of
  ephedra products sold as mood-
  altering substances. But the law does
  not ban ephedra products sold for
  other reasons.

- In 1996 New York banned the sale of twenty ephedra products made for getting high. Store owners who sell them face a $2,000 fine and a year in prison. But the sale of ephedra products for weight loss or body building is still legal. So is the sale of drugs for colds, asthma, flu, and allergies.

Sellers Against Herbal Stimulants

Some store owners didn't wait for new state laws. They stopped selling certain herbal stimulants on their own. Fresh Fields, a large chain of health-food supermarkets, is an example. It no longer sells supplements that carry unproven claims. That includes products with pennyroyal, comfrey, yohimbe, kola nut, and ephedra.

Even herb makers are being more careful. The American Herbal Products Association is made up of many herb companies. In 1994 it asked its members to temporarily stop selling comfrey and chaparral or to put warning labels on them.

What Lies Ahead

Many people feel that stricter herbal laws are needed in the United States. In 1996 a new bill was introduced in Congress.

It would classify ephedra products for getting high as drugs. If it passes, those products would then be controlled by the FDA. They would have to be tested for safety before being sold.

Others believe that in the future, *all* herbal products will be classified as drugs.

CHAPTER 6

Getting Help

*T*housands of teenagers abuse herbal stimulants. Many have been hurt by them. Some have even died. You may be a user yourself. Or you may be thinking about using them.

Before taking an herbal stimulant—for *any* reason—get advice from an expert. Who can you turn to? Here are some suggestions.

Your Doctor

Your family doctor probably knows more about herbal stimulants than anyone else you know. Many doctors give them to patients. They know how herbs affect the body. They also know if an herb is safe or unsafe.

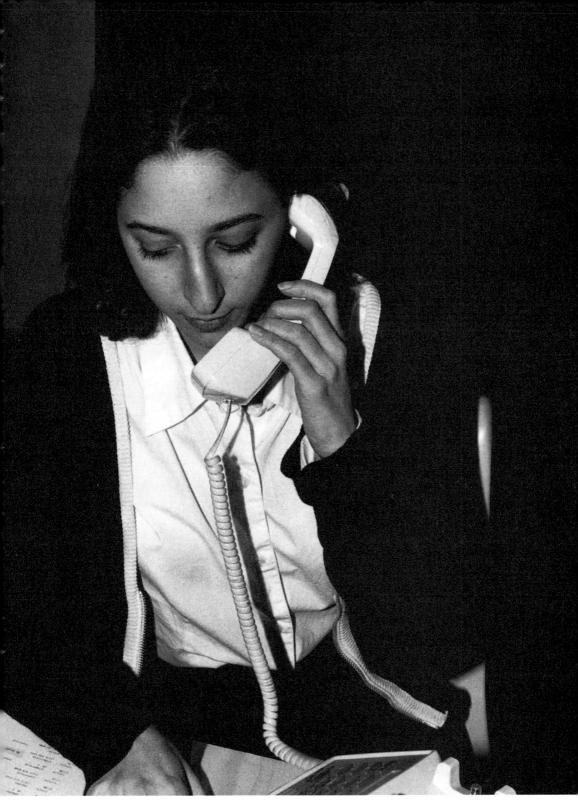
There are many resources you can contact if you want more information about herbal stimulants.

54 You may want to take an herbal stimulant to lose weight or build muscles. Your
doctor knows your medical history. Ask
what the herbs can do to *your* body. If
your doctor approves the product for you,
learn how much you should take and how
often.

It is important to take good care of
yourself. The more you know about what
you put into your body—be it an herb or
a medicine—the better. In the end, it
could save your life.

A Drug Clinic or Hot Line

Your city or town probably has a drug-
abuse clinic. The local telephone book
can help you find it. Look in the
Yellow Pages under "Drug Abuse." Or
call the local hospital and ask where it is.
Then pay a visit. The staff there will be
glad to share information on herbal
stimulants.

Your School Counselor

Many school counselors are trained to
know about herbal stimulants. They may
have dealt with other students who take
them. Your counselor can warn you of
problems that stimulants have caused
other students.

Your Teacher

You may feel most at ease talking with a teacher you like and trust. Ask your teacher if you can speak to him or her confidentially. Teachers might not be experts on herbal stimulants. But they can tell you where to find the answers you need.

Your Parents

If you now take herbal stimulants or are thinking about it, your parents can help. They may already know something about the subject.

It isn't always easy to start a conversation like this with them. You might begin by telling them about this book. Tell what you've learned about herbal stimulants. Then say what's on your mind. Speak sincerely, and you may be surprised. Your parents will probably be glad to help you as best they can.

Yourself

That's right. If you're not willing to talk to others, at least rely on yourself. Learn all you can about herbal stimulants. Reading this book is a good start. Then go to your school or local library. Find

56 other books, magazines, and newspaper articles.

If you still plan to take herbal stimulants, remember these rules:

- *Never* take herbal products if you're on medication, unless you first check with a doctor.
- Don't take herbal products if you have a condition like diabetes, high blood pressure, or allergies. Check with a doctor first.
- If you're pregnant or nursing a baby, never take herbal products without a doctor's okay. And never give herbal products to a baby without checking, too.
- If you feel any pain, dizziness, nausea, or other bad effects, stop taking the product. Call a doctor immediately.
- Be sure to take the herb in its proper form. Swallowing an herb that's meant to be rubbed on the skin can be fatal.
- Always take the product in the amount suggested on the package. Never take more than that.
- If no amounts are suggested, always start with a very small dosage.

- Check the package carefully for warnings of possible dangers or side effects.

- Look for labels that warn against taking the herbal product in combination with particular foods. An herbal stimulant by itself may not harm you. But together with certain foods, it may be dangerous or deadly.
- Don't take advice from people who aren't experts. Store clerks, fitness trainers, and friends don't always know what they're talking about.
- Stay away from products that mix two or more herbs. Herbs can be mixed in a deadly combination.
- Stay away from any product that claims to cure everything.
- Look for the word *standardized* on the package. That means the maker has adjusted the chemicals so that each dose is a safe amount. Also look for labels that say "FDA Approved."
- Above all, if you use herbal stimulants, don't overdo it. Too much of *anything* can be harmful.

Glossary—
Explaining New Words

abuse To use a drug or herb in a way that it is not meant to be used.

additive Something added to a food, such as for flavor, color, or preserving.

asthma A condition involving wheezing, coughing, and difficulty in breathing.

caffeine A chemical stimulant found in herbs such as coffee, tea, and kola.

contaminated Spoiled or made harmful through contact with something else.

dosage The amount of a medicine taken at one time; same as *dose*.

extract A concentrated form of an herb or food.

hepatitis A disease in which the liver becomes inflamed.

herb A plant whose leaves, flowers, fruits, bark, or stem is used for medicine.

herbalist One who grows, collects, or works with herbs.

herbal medicine The practice of using herbs to cure illness.

impotence A condition in which a male cannot get an erection to have sex.

insomnia A condition in which it is hard for someone to fall or stay asleep.

pharmacist A person who is licensed to prepare and sell drugs or other medicines.

pharmacy A drugstore.

preservative Something added to food to keep it from spoiling.

substance A particular kind of matter or chemical makeup.

supplement Something added to improve one's diet, such as an herb or vitamin.

synthetic Made by a person, rather than being in natural form.

tincture A substance in a solution of alcohol or water and alcohol.

Where to Go for Help

American Council for Drug Education
204 Monroe Street
Rockville, MD 20852
(800) 488-DRUG

American Herbal Products Association
4733 Bethesda Avenue
Suite 345
Bethesda, MD 20814
(512) 469-6355

DARE America, Inc.
P.O. Box 2090
Los Angeles, CA 90051-0090
(310) 215-0575
(800) 223-3273

e-mail address: dare@flash.net

Food and Drug Administration Office of Consumer Affairs
1500 Fishers Lane
Rockville, MD 20857
FDA Consumer Inquiries Line
(800) 332-1088

The Herb Research Foundation
1007 Pearl Street Suite 200
Boulder, CO 80302
(303) 449-2265
(800) 748-2617
e-mail address: info@herbs.org

National Clearinghouse for Alcohol and Drug Information
P.O. Box 2345
Rockville, MD 20852
(800) 729-6686
Web site: http://www.health.org

Natural Health & Longevity Resource Center
Web site: http://www.all-natural.com

For Further Reading

Ball, Jacqueline A. *Everything You Need to Know About Drug Abuse*. Rev. ed. New York: Rosen Publishing Group, 1994.

Berger, Gilda & Berger, Melvin. *Drug Abuse A-Z*. New York: Enslow Publishers, 1990.

Castleman, Michael. *The Healing Herbs*: *The Ultimate Guide to the Curative Power of Nature's Medicines*. Emmaus, PA: Rodale Press, 1991.

Myers, Arthur. *Drugs and Peer Pressure*. New York: Rosen Publishing Group, 1995.

Tyler, Varro E. *Honest Herbal*: *A Sensible Guide to the Use of Herbs and Related Remedies*. Philadelphia, PA: Hayworth Press, 1993.

Index

About the Author

Meish Goldish is the author of more than thirty fiction and nonfiction books for children and young adults. A former high school English teacher, he visits many elementary and high school classrooms annually to talk about writing. He is an avid theatergoer who also performs his own one-man musical show. He currently lives in Teaneck, NJ.

Photo Credits

Cover photo: Ira Fox
Photo on page 23: Kathleen McClancy. All other photos: Ira Fox.